M000250208

THIS PLANNER
Belongs To:

_____

DEDICATION

This book is dedicated to all the brave survivors who are battling and living with mental health issues that deserve to be happy.

Your are my inspiration for producing books and I'm honored to be a part of keeping all your mental health notes and discoveries all in one place.

This journal notebook will help you record your details, thoughts, feelings, emotions, etc while dealing with your own personal battle.

Thoughtfully put together with these sections to record: About Me, Coping Strategies, Anxiety & Mood Charts, Gratitude & Happiness Tracker, Trigger Tracker, Self Improvement, Daily Reflection & Awareness, Post Therapy Chart and much, much more.

HOW TO USE THIS BOOK:

The purpose of this book is to keep all of your mindfulness writings all in one place. It will help keep you organized.

This Mental Health Journal will allow you to accurately document triggers, findings, etc. It's a great way to chart your course through all of your thoughts and feelings.

Here are examples of the prompts for you to fill in and write about yourself in this book:

1. About Me - A self discovery section to find out more about yourself.

2. Coping Strategies - You will want to write down & track the different ways you feel about yourself so you can better manage and cope with self-doubt and negative feelings that keep you down.

3. Anxiety Level Chart - Color the boxes on the chart to rate your level of anxiety when you face certain situations.

4. Gratitude & Happiness Tracker - Spend some time self reflecting & focus your thoughts on the joys in your life.

5. Mood Chart - The mood wheel chart can be used to record your positive, negative and neutral emotions every month.

6. Life Assessment - Focus on areas in your life that you would like to be better and ways to improve it.

7. Trigger Tracker - Tracking your experiences that generate negative thoughts and emotions.

8. Self Improvement - What are your self sabotaging habits and ways to work on them.

9. Daily Reflection & Daily Awareness - Take a moment each day focusing on your day, highlights, gratefulness, mood, happiness, challenges. Chart your good days and your bad days.

10. Post Therapy Chart - Notes from your therapy session.

11. Weekly Assessment & Reflections - Overview of your week.

DATE:

ALL ABOUT *me*

1. What are you most grateful for in your life?

Keeping track of what you're most grateful for will keep you focused on the blessings in your life. Consider the many reasons you have to be grateful BELOW:

2. What do you love about yourself?

Self love isn't always easy but writing down what you're most proud of will help clear your mind of the criticism and negativity you may feel.

3. Where is your happy place?

Where do you feel most at peace? Do you have a favorite spot that allows you to refocus your energy, find inner peace and feel happiness? Describe your happy place.

ALL ABOUT me

4. What do you enjoy doing?

What are your favorite activities where you are able to boost your mood and free your mind? This could be a hobby or physical activity, or perhaps something entirely different.

5. Who can you rely on?

Describe the people in your life that you can count on when things get tough. Who do you feel closest to?

6. How can you improve your life?

What changes can you make that will ultimately improve your life and give you joy? This could be career or personal related. Please share your thoughts below.

ALL ABOUT me

7. My greatest accomplishments are:

What are some of the things you are most proud of?

8. What do you wish others knew about you?

What do you wish others knew about who you really are? What do you feel others overlook?

9. What are your greatest aspirations?

Whether it be personal, career or family goals, list them below.

DEAR FUTURE *Self...*

FOCUS ON YOUR VISION OF A HAPPY FUTURE

FAMILY GOALS

CAREER GOALS

SELF CARE

RELATIONSHIP

HEALTH GOALS

FRIENDSHIPS

PERSONAL

FINANCIAL

TRAVEL

PASSIONS

NEW SKILLS

OTHER

5 YEARS FROM NOW

10 YEARS FROM NOW

COPING *Strategies*

Write down the different ways you feel about yourself as well as personal situations, and how you can better manage and cope with self-doubt and negative feelings.

WHEN I'M FEELING...	I WILL MANAGE IT BY...

WHEN I'M FEELING...	I WILL MANAGE IT BY...

WHEN I'M FEELING...	I WILL MANAGE IT BY...

WHEN I'M FEELING...	I WILL MANAGE IT BY...

WHEN I'M FEELING...	I WILL MANAGE IT BY...

WHEN I'M FEELING...	I WILL MANAGE IT BY...

WHEN I'M FEELING...	I WILL MANAGE IT BY...

OTHER IDEAS / NOTES

DATE:

ANXIETY *debrief*

Describe a situation where you felt anxious:

What were the physical symptoms you experienced?

Did you face the situation or remove yourself from it?

How did you cope with this anxiety? Do you believe your thoughts and reactions were rational?

ANXIETY *levels*

Use the chart below to rate your level of anxiety when facing various situations by coloring the boxes:

SITUATION: Meeting Someone New

ANXIETY LEVEL

DO YOU: Face this fear   Avoid this situation

SITUATION: Going to the grocery store

ANXIETY LEVEL

DO YOU: Face this fear   Avoid this situation

SITUATION: Stating your opinion when potentially controversial or opposing.

ANXIETY LEVEL

DO YOU: Face this fear   Avoid this situation

SITUATION: Stand up for yourself when treated unfairly or poorly.

ANXIETY LEVEL

DO YOU: Face this fear   Avoid this situation

SITUATION: Spending time alone with friends and/or family.

ANXIETY LEVEL

DO YOU: Face this fear   Avoid this situation

SITUATION: Being watched/observed when doing something/completing a task or activity.

ANXIETY LEVEL

DO YOU: Face this fear   Avoid this situation

UNDERSTANDING *anxiety*

Understanding the origin of your anxiety will help you learn new ways to manage your responses.

SITUATION: Meeting Someone New

WHAT IS YOUR BIGGEST FEAR WHEN FACING THIS SITUATION?

SITUATION: Going to the grocery store

WHAT IS YOUR BIGGEST FEAR WHEN FACING THIS SITUATION?

SITUATION: Stating your opinion.

WHAT IS YOUR BIGGEST FEAR WHEN FACING THIS SITUATION?

SITUATION: Stand up for yourself.

WHAT IS YOUR BIGGEST FEAR WHEN FACING THIS SITUATION?

SITUATION: Spending time alone with friends.

WHAT IS YOUR BIGGEST FEAR WHEN FACING THIS SITUATION?

SITUATION: Being watched/observed.

WHAT IS YOUR BIGGEST FEAR WHEN FACING THIS SITUATION?

GRATEFUL *Life*

What are the things you are most grateful for? Spend time self-reflecting on the many blessings in your life. Shift your focus on gratitude and rid yourself of negative emotions and toxic thoughts.

1	2	3
4	5	6
7	8	9
10	11	12

HAPPINESS Is...

Complete the following sentences to refocus your mind on the joys in your life:

I FEEL MOST RELAXED WHEN:

I AM LESS STRESSED WHEN:

MY STRENGTHS ARE:

I AM A GOOD FRIEND BECAUSE:

I AM MOST EXCITED BY:

I AM MOST FOCUSED WHEN:

I FEEL MOST APPRECIATED WHEN:

I AM MOST MOTIVATED WHEN:

THOUGHTS *Tracker*

MONDAY'S THOUGHTS

TUESDAY'S THOUGHTS

WEDNESDAY'S THOUGHTS

THURSDAY'S THOUGHTS

FRIDAY'S THOUGHTS

SATURDAY'S THOUGHTS

SUNDAY'S THOUGHTS

TRANSFORMING *Thoughts*

TRANSFORMING NEGATIVE THOUGHTS

We all deal with negative thoughts and self-doubt. Use this space to keep track of those feelings and focus on how you can replace them with positive thoughts that promote self-growth.

NEGATIVE THOUGHT	REPLACEMENT THOUGHT
NEGATIVE THOUGHT	REPLACEMENT THOUGHT
NEGATIVE THOUGHT	REPLACEMENT THOUGHT
NEGATIVE THOUGHT	REPLACEMENT THOUGHT
NEGATIVE THOUGHT	REPLACEMENT THOUGHT
NEGATIVE THOUGHT	REPLACEMENT THOUGHT

PERSONAL REFLECTIONS

SELF AWARENESS *Chart*

CHALLENGE NEGATIVE THOUGHTS AND FEELINGS

It's easy to get lost in our own headspace so it's important that you question any negative feelings so you can sort through your emotions effectively. Use this worksheet to document your progress.

THOUGHT

IS THE THOUGHT VALID?

HOW DO YOU REACT TO THIS NEGATIVE THOUGHT?

WHAT COULD YOU DO TO AVOID FEELING THIS WAY?

THOUGHTS & REFLECTIONS

MOOD Chart

Use the wheel below to document your moods every month.
Use 3 different colors to represent positive, negative or neutral emotions.

POSITIVE   NEGATIVE   NEUTRAL

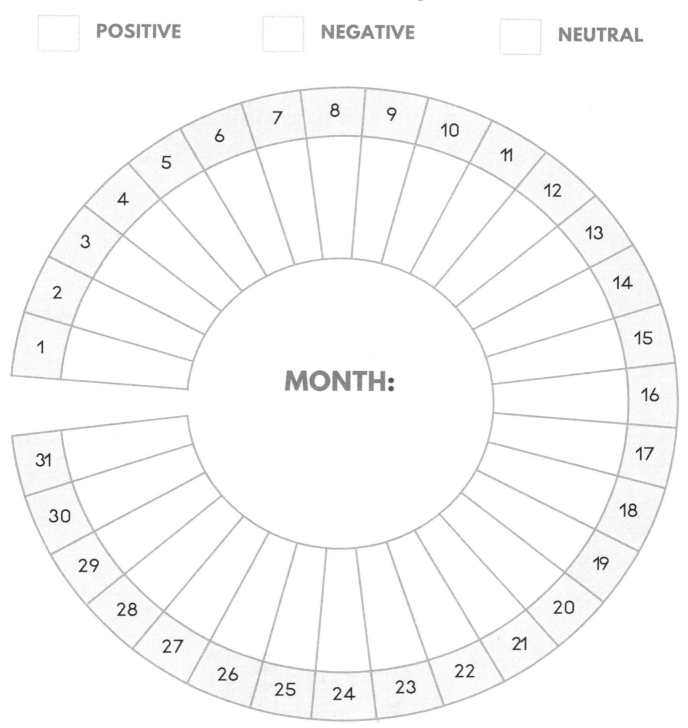

MONTH:

SLEEP *Tracker*

MONTH: _____

Sleep plays a major factor in our ability to cope with anxiety and depression. Keep track of your sleep pattern in order to determine how the amount of rest may be affecting your mental health.

DAY	HOURS SLEPT	QUALITY OF SLEEP	THOUGHTS
1			
2			
3			
4			
5			
6			
7			
8			
9			
10			
11			
12			
13			
14			
15			
16			
17			
18			
19			
20			
21			
22			
23			
24			
25			
26			
27			
28			
29			
30			
31			

LIFE Assessment

SUMMARIZE HOW YOU **FEEL** ABOUT YOUR LIFE

TOP 3 AREAS OF YOUR LIFE YOU'D LIKE TO **IMPROVE**

01

02

03

3 WAYS YOU CAN **ACCOMPLISH** YOUR LIFE GOALS

TRIGGER *Tracker*

Keep track of experiences that generate negative thoughts and emotions.

DATE	INCIDENT	REACTION

GRATEFUL *Heart*

DAY	TODAY I AM GRATEFUL FOR:
1	
2	
3	
4	
5	
6	
7	
8	
9	
10	
11	
12	
13	
14	
15	
16	
17	
18	
19	
20	
21	
22	
23	
24	
25	
26	
27	
28	
29	
30	
31	

SELF Improvement

WHAT ARE YOUR SELF SABOTAGE HABITS?

Eliminate Negative Habits

≫
≫
≫
≫
≫
≫

Create Positive Habits

HOW CAN YOU IMPROVE YOUR MENTAL HEALTH?

What Key Areas Need Work?

≫
≫
≫
≫
≫
≫

What Are Some Steps You Can Take?

ANALYZING THE PEOPLE IN YOUR LIFE

Who Are The Negative Influences?

≫
≫
≫
≫
≫
≫

Who Are The Positive Influences?

HOW DO I HOLD MYSELF ACCOUNTABLE?

What I Know I'm Responsible For

≫
≫
≫
≫
≫

Who Helps Keep Me Accountable?

SELF CARE *Ideas*

NURTURE YOUR MIND

Discover new hobbies

Read a book

Take a road trip

Keep a journal

Talk to a friend

Follow inspiring people

Challenge yourself

Be grateful

Call an old friend

Try something new

FEED YOUR SPIRIT

Have "me-time"

Listen to music

Read poetry

Write "future-self"

Paint

Meditate

TAKE CARE OF YOUR BODY

Eat healthy

Start a workout plan

Get enough sleep

Stay hydrated

Yoga

Ideas

SELF CARE *Planner*

Self-care involves taking care of yourself emotionally, mentally and physically.
Create a self-care plan by adding activities to the categories below.

MENTAL SELF-CARE

_____
_____
_____
_____

PHYSICAL SELF-CARE (GET ACTIVE)

_____
_____
_____
_____

EMOTIONAL SELF-CARE

_____
_____
_____
_____

DAILY HABITS (SLEEP, ETC.)

_____
_____
_____
_____

REACH OUT (SOCIALIZE)

_____
_____
_____
_____

SUPPORT NETWORK

_____
_____
_____
_____

OTHER:

_____
_____
_____
_____
_____
_____
_____
_____

SELF CARE Tracker

Self care is an important step in managing anxiety and depression. It helps us recharge, reset and nurtures our mind and soul. Focus on incorporating one self-care activity into your daily life.

THOUGHT *Log*

Keep track of negative thoughts so you can learn how to control irrational responses and triggers.

DATE	INCIDENT	INITIAL REACTION	RATIONAL REACTION

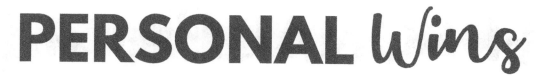

PERSONAL Wins

MONTH:

It's important to celebrate both minor and major wins when it comes to your mental health and the coping strategies you've learned along the way. You've come a long way!

2 RECENT WINS

TOP 3 MILESTONES

1
2
3

3 THINGS I'VE LEARNED ABOUT MYSELF OVER THE LAST YEAR

PERSONAL REFLECTIONS	HOW I'VE LEARNED TO COPE WITH EMOTIONS

NOTES

PERSONAL *Rewards*

MONTH:

Make sure to reward yourself for accomplishments throughout your journey.
Whether it's a visit to your favorite restaurant, a bubble bath or an evening with friends, it's
important to celebrate your progress every step of the way.

IDEAS FOR PERSONAL REWARDS

1	2
3	4
5	6

HOW I FELT BEFORE	HOW I REWARDED MYSELF	HOW I FELT AFTER REWARD

NOTES	PERSONAL REFLECTIONS/THOUGHTS

ANXIETY *Tracker*

Document the days when you experienced anxiety. This page includes a 3-week tracker.

ANXIETY LEVELS (1-MILD, 10 SEVERE)

														NOTES:
MON	01	02	03	04	05	06	07	08	09	10	11	12		
TUE	01	02	03	04	05	06	07	08	09	10	11	12		
WED	01	02	03	04	05	06	07	08	09	10	11	12		
THU	01	02	03	04	05	06	07	08	09	10	11	12		
FRI	01	02	03	04	05	06	07	08	09	10	11	12		
SAT	01	02	03	04	05	06	07	08	09	10	11	12		
SUN	01	02	03	04	05	06	07	08	09	10	11	12		
MON	01	02	03	04	05	06	07	08	09	10	11	12		
TUE	01	02	03	04	05	06	07	08	09	10	11	12		
WED	01	02	03	04	05	06	07	08	09	10	11	12		
THU	01	02	03	04	05	06	07	08	09	10	11	12		
FRI	01	02	03	04	05	06	07	08	09	10	11	12		
SAT	01	02	03	04	05	06	07	08	09	10	11	12		
SUN	01	02	03	04	05	06	07	08	09	10	11	12		
MON	01	02	03	04	05	06	07	08	09	10	11	12		
TUE	01	02	03	04	05	06	07	08	09	10	11	12		
WED	01	02	03	04	05	06	07	08	09	10	11	12		
THU	01	02	03	04	05	06	07	08	09	10	11	12		
FRI	01	02	03	04	05	06	07	08	09	10	11	12		
SAT	01	02	03	04	05	06	07	08	09	10	11	12		
SUN	01	02	03	04	05	06	07	08	09	10	11	12		

DATE I STARTED TRACKING:

DEPRESSION *Tracker*

Document the days when you experienced depression. This page includes a 3-week tracker.

DEPRESSION LEVELS (1-MILD, 10 SEVERE)

MON	01	02	03	04	05	06	07	08	09	10	11	12
TUE	01	02	03	04	05	06	07	08	09	10	11	12
WED	01	02	03	04	05	06	07	08	09	10	11	12
THU	01	02	03	04	05	06	07	08	09	10	11	12
FRI	01	02	03	04	05	06	07	08	09	10	11	12
SAT	01	02	03	04	05	06	07	08	09	10	11	12
SUN	01	02	03	04	05	06	07	08	09	10	11	12
MON	01	02	03	04	05	06	07	08	09	10	11	12
TUE	01	02	03	04	05	06	07	08	09	10	11	12
WED	01	02	03	04	05	06	07	08	09	10	11	12
THU	01	02	03	04	05	06	07	08	09	10	11	12
FRI	01	02	03	04	05	06	07	08	09	10	11	12
SAT	01	02	03	04	05	06	07	08	09	10	11	12
SUN	01	02	03	04	05	06	07	08	09	10	11	12
MON	01	02	03	04	05	06	07	08	09	10	11	12
TUE	01	02	03	04	05	06	07	08	09	10	11	12
WED	01	02	03	04	05	06	07	08	09	10	11	12
THU	01	02	03	04	05	06	07	08	09	10	11	12
FRI	01	02	03	04	05	06	07	08	09	10	11	12
SAT	01	02	03	04	05	06	07	08	09	10	11	12
SUN	01	02	03	04	05	06	07	08	09	10	11	12

NOTES:

DATE I STARTED TRACKING:

RESET *your mind*

We can't always control the way our thoughts but we can learn to transform negative feelings into positive ones and control our reactions and impulses. Use the chart below to start the process.

WHEN I FEEL LIKE:

I WILL TRY TO CONTROL BY REACTIONS BY:

}
}
}
}
}
}
}
}
}
}
}
}

NOTES & REFLECTIONS

DOODLES & SCRIBBLES

LOVE *Yourself*

STEP 1: MAKE YOURSELF A PRIORITY

It's important to always put yourself first by listening to your inner voice. Let it guide you in eliminating toxic people and negative sources. Don't be afraid to distance yourself from people and places that make you feel unhappy or who don't support your journey.

STEP 2: FACE YOUR FEARS

Don't be afraid to confront your fears and self-doubt. Why do you feel unworthy at times? What are you most worried about?

STEP 3: BE ACCOUNTABLE

Hold yourself accountable for the things you can control and change. There are things in your life only you can change.

STEP 4: FORGIVE YOURSELF

Let go of past mistakes – you can't go back in time. We all have regrets and while it's important to hold yourself accountable for mistakes, you can only truly heal when you learn to forgive yourself. Free your mind so it can focus on a better you and a happier tomorrow.

STEP 5: ACCEPT WHERE YOU ARE IN YOUR JOURNEY

Don't allow yourself to grow frustrated that you aren't able to race towards the finish line. Your journey will take time so give yourself permission to fail while also learning to accept where you are right now. Take it one day at a time. You owe it to yourself to stay focused on the road ahead while celebrating every milestone along the way.

Write down your thoughts, reflections and ideas below:

Thoughts

SELF CARE *Focus*

TOP 3 SELF-CARE ACTIVITIES

HOW THEY MAKE ME FEEL

OTHER SELF-CARE ACTIVITIES THAT MAKE ME HAPPY

01

02

03

FAVORITE QUOTES/WORDS OF ENCOURAGEMENT

TRIGGER *Sources*

Discover what causes emotional pain and negative thoughts in your life.

Describe the negative reaction/response you would like to overcome:

Consider the aspects of your life below and write down how each category can cause the above trigger.

PERSONAL

PEOPLE

PLACES

SITUATIONS

Think about the different ways you can overcome your triggers when dealing with each category.
How can you better control your reactions and manage frustrating situations?

HAPPINESS Tracker

Keep track of how often you feel happy and calm and what you did to minimize negative responses.

DATE:

HAPPINESS RATING: ☆☆☆☆☆

DATE:

HAPPINESS RATING: ☆☆☆☆☆

DATE:

HAPPINESS RATING: ☆☆☆☆☆

DATE:

HAPPINESS RATING: ☆☆☆☆☆

DATE:

HAPPINESS RATING: ☆☆☆☆☆

DATE:

HAPPINESS RATING: ☆☆☆☆☆

DAILY *Reflection*

DATE:

HOW I FEEL TODAY

MY GREATEST CHALLENGE

MOOD TRACKER:

MORNING:

EVENING:

I FELT HAPPY WHEN:

I FELT EXCITED WHEN:

I FELT ENERGIZED WHEN:

Today's Highlights

What I'm Grateful For Today

DAILY *Awareness*

MONTH:

M	T	W	T	F	S	S
☐	☐	☐	☐	☐	☐	☐

HOW I'M FEELING TODAY

3 WORDS TO DESCRIBE MY DAY

STRUGGLES

HIGHLIGHT OF MY DAY

DAILY ACCOMPLISHMENTS

DAILY Reflection

DATE:

HOW I FEEL TODAY

MY GREATEST CHALLENGE

MOOD TRACKER:

MORNING:

EVENING:

I FELT HAPPY WHEN:

I FELT EXCITED WHEN:

I FELT ENERGIZED WHEN:

Today's Highlights

What I'm Grateful For Today

DAILY *Awareness*

MONTH:

M	T	W	T	F	S	S
☐	☐	☐	☐	☐	☐	☐

HOW I'M FEELING TODAY

3 WORDS TO DESCRIBE MY DAY

STRUGGLES

HIGHLIGHT OF MY DAY

DAILY ACCOMPLISHMENTS

DATE:

DAILY *Reflection*

HOW I FEEL TODAY

MY GREATEST CHALLENGE

MOOD TRACKER:

MORNING:

EVENING:

I FELT HAPPY WHEN:

I FELT EXCITED WHEN:

I FELT ENERGIZED WHEN:

Today's Highlights

What I'm Grateful For Today

DAILY *Awareness*

MONTH:

M	T	W	T	F	S	S
☐	☐	☐	☐	☐	☐	☐

HOW I'M FEELING TODAY

3 WORDS TO DESCRIBE MY DAY

STRUGGLES

HIGHLIGHT OF MY DAY

DAILY ACCOMPLISHMENTS

DATE:

DAILY *Reflection*

HOW I FEEL TODAY

MY GREATEST CHALLENGE

MOOD TRACKER:

MORNING:

EVENING:

I FELT HAPPY WHEN:

I FELT EXCITED WHEN:

I FELT ENERGIZED WHEN:

Today's Highlights

What I'm Grateful For Today

DAILY Awareness

MONTH: _____

M T W T F S S
☐ ☐ ☐ ☐ ☐ ☐ ☐

HOW I'M FEELING TODAY

3 WORDS TO DESCRIBE MY DAY

STRUGGLES

HIGHLIGHT OF MY DAY

DAILY ACCOMPLISHMENTS

DATE:

DAILY *Reflection*

HOW I FEEL TODAY

MY GREATEST CHALLENGE

MOOD TRACKER:

MORNING:

EVENING:

I FELT HAPPY WHEN:

I FELT EXCITED WHEN:

I FELT ENERGIZED WHEN:

Today's Highlights

What I'm Grateful For Today

DAILY *Awareness*

MONTH:

M	T	W	T	F	S	S
☐	☐	☐	☐	☐	☐	☐

HOW I'M FEELING TODAY

3 WORDS TO DESCRIBE MY DAY

STRUGGLES

HIGHLIGHT OF MY DAY

DAILY ACCOMPLISHMENTS

DATE:

DAILY *Reflection*

HOW I FEEL TODAY

MY GREATEST CHALLENGE

MOOD TRACKER:

MORNING:

EVENING:

I FELT HAPPY WHEN:

I FELT EXCITED WHEN:

I FELT ENERGIZED WHEN:

Today's Highlights

What I'm Grateful For Today

DAILY *Awareness*

MONTH:

M	T	W	T	F	S	S
☐	☐	☐	☐	☐	☐	☐

HOW I'M FEELING TODAY

3 WORDS TO DESCRIBE MY DAY

STRUGGLES

HIGHLIGHT OF MY DAY

DAILY ACCOMPLISHMENTS

DATE:

DAILY *Reflection*

HOW I FEEL TODAY

MY GREATEST CHALLENGE

MOOD TRACKER:

MORNING:

EVENING:

I FELT HAPPY WHEN:

I FELT EXCITED WHEN:

I FELT ENERGIZED WHEN:

Today's Highlights

What I'm Grateful For Today

DAILY *Awareness*

MONTH:

M	T	W	T	F	S	S
☐	☐	☐	☐	☐	☐	☐

HOW I'M FEELING TODAY

3 WORDS TO DESCRIBE MY DAY

STRUGGLES

HIGHLIGHT OF MY DAY

DAILY ACCOMPLISHMENTS

POST Therapy Chart

DATE:

SUMMARY/OVERVIEW OF THERAPY SESSION

WHAT WE DISCUSSED

HOW IT MADE ME FEEL

WHAT I LEARNED

WHAT I WANT TO DISCUSS NEXT

Rate your session to keep track of progress.

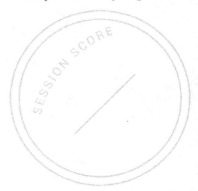

SESSION SCORE

WEEKLY *Assessment*

	SLEEP	MOOD	POSITIVES	NEGATIVES
MONDAY				
TUESDAY				
WEDNESDAY				
THURSDAY				
FRIDAY				
SATURADY				
SUNDAY				

WEEKLY *Reflections*

Monday

Tuesday

Wednesday

Thursday

Friday

Saturday

Sunday

DATE:

DAILY *Reflection*

HOW I FEEL TODAY

MY GREATEST CHALLENGE

MOOD TRACKER:

MORNING:

EVENING:

I FELT HAPPY WHEN:

I FELT EXCITED WHEN:

I FELT ENERGIZED WHEN:

Today's Highlights

What I'm Grateful For Today

DAILY *Awareness*

MONTH:

M	T	W	T	F	S	S
☐	☐	☐	☐	☐	☐	☐

HOW I'M FEELING TODAY

3 WORDS TO DESCRIBE MY DAY

STRUGGLES

HIGHLIGHT OF MY DAY

DAILY ACCOMPLISHMENTS

DAILY *Reflection*

HOW I FEEL TODAY

MY GREATEST CHALLENGE

MOOD TRACKER:

MORNING:

EVENING:

I FELT HAPPY WHEN:

I FELT EXCITED WHEN:

I FELT ENERGIZED WHEN:

Today's Highlights

What I'm Grateful For Today

DAILY *Awareness*

MONTH:

M	T	W	T	F	S	S
☐	☐	☐	☐	☐	☐	☐

HOW I'M FEELING TODAY

3 WORDS TO DESCRIBE MY DAY

STRUGGLES

HIGHLIGHT OF MY DAY

DAILY ACCOMPLISHMENTS

DATE:

DAILY *Reflection*

HOW I FEEL TODAY

MY GREATEST CHALLENGE

MOOD TRACKER:

MORNING:

EVENING:

I FELT HAPPY WHEN:

I FELT EXCITED WHEN:

I FELT ENERGIZED WHEN:

Today's Highlights

What I'm Grateful For Today

DAILY *Awareness*

MONTH:

M T W T F S S
☐ ☐ ☐ ☐ ☐ ☐ ☐

HOW I'M FEELING TODAY

3 WORDS TO DESCRIBE MY DAY

STRUGGLES

HIGHLIGHT OF MY DAY

DAILY ACCOMPLISHMENTS

DAILY *Reflection*

HOW I FEEL TODAY

MY GREATEST CHALLENGE

MOOD TRACKER:

MORNING:

EVENING:

I FELT HAPPY WHEN:

I FELT EXCITED WHEN:

I FELT ENERGIZED WHEN:

Today's Highlights

What I'm Grateful For Today

DAILY *Awareness*

MONTH:

M	T	W	T	F	S	S
☐	☐	☐	☐	☐	☐	☐

HOW I'M FEELING TODAY

3 WORDS TO DESCRIBE MY DAY

STRUGGLES

HIGHLIGHT OF MY DAY

DAILY ACCOMPLISHMENTS

DATE:

DAILY *Reflection*

HOW I FEEL TODAY

MY GREATEST CHALLENGE

MOOD TRACKER:

MORNING:

EVENING:

I FELT HAPPY WHEN:

I FELT EXCITED WHEN:

I FELT ENERGIZED WHEN:

Today's Highlights

What I'm Grateful For Today

DAILY *Awareness*

MONTH:

M	T	W	T	F	S	S
☐	☐	☐	☐	☐	☐	☐

HOW I'M FEELING TODAY

3 WORDS TO DESCRIBE MY DAY

STRUGGLES

HIGHLIGHT OF MY DAY

DAILY ACCOMPLISHMENTS

DAILY Reflection

HOW I FEEL TODAY

MY GREATEST CHALLENGE

MOOD TRACKER:

MORNING:

EVENING:

I FELT HAPPY WHEN:

I FELT EXCITED WHEN:

I FELT ENERGIZED WHEN:

Today's Highlights

What I'm Grateful For Today

DAILY *Awareness*

MONTH: _____

M T W T F S S
☐ ☐ ☐ ☐ ☐ ☐ ☐

HOW I'M FEELING TODAY

3 WORDS TO DESCRIBE MY DAY

STRUGGLES

HIGHLIGHT OF MY DAY

DAILY ACCOMPLISHMENTS

DATE:

DAILY *Reflection*

HOW I FEEL TODAY

MY GREATEST CHALLENGE

MOOD TRACKER:

MORNING:

EVENING:

I FELT HAPPY WHEN:

I FELT EXCITED WHEN:

I FELT ENERGIZED WHEN:

Today's Highlights

What I'm Grateful For Today

DAILY *Awareness*

MONTH:

M	T	W	T	F	S	S
☐	☐	☐	☐	☐	☐	☐

HOW I'M FEELING TODAY

3 WORDS TO DESCRIBE MY DAY

STRUGGLES

HIGHLIGHT OF MY DAY

DAILY ACCOMPLISHMENTS

POST *Therapy Chart*

DATE:

SUMMARY/OVERVIEW OF THERAPY SESSION

WHAT WE DISCUSSED

HOW IT MADE ME FEEL

WHAT I LEARNED

WHAT I WANT TO DISCUSS NEXT

Rate your session to
keep track of progress.

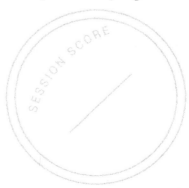

SESSION SCORE

WEEKLY *Assessment*

	SLEEP	MOOD	POSITIVES	NEGATIVES
MONDAY				
TUESDAY				
WEDNESDAY				
THURSDAY				
FRIDAY				
SATURADY				
SUNDAY				

WEEKLY *Reflections*

Monday

Tuesday

Wednesday

Thursday

Friday

Saturday

Sunday

DAILY *Reflection*

DATE: ___

HOW I FEEL TODAY

MY GREATEST CHALLENGE

MOOD TRACKER:

MORNING: ___

EVENING: ___

I FELT HAPPY WHEN:

I FELT EXCITED WHEN:

I FELT ENERGIZED WHEN:

Today's Highlights

What I'm Grateful For Today

DAILY *Awareness*

MONTH:

M	T	W	T	F	S	S
☐	☐	☐	☐	☐	☐	☐

HOW I'M FEELING TODAY

3 WORDS TO DESCRIBE MY DAY

STRUGGLES

HIGHLIGHT OF MY DAY

DAILY ACCOMPLISHMENTS

DATE:

DAILY *Reflection*

HOW I FEEL TODAY

MY GREATEST CHALLENGE

MOOD TRACKER:

MORNING:

EVENING:

I FELT HAPPY WHEN:

I FELT EXCITED WHEN:

I FELT ENERGIZED WHEN:

Today's Highlights

What I'm Grateful For Today

DAILY *Awareness*

MONTH:

M	T	W	T	F	S	S
☐	☐	☐	☐	☐	☐	☐

HOW I'M FEELING TODAY

3 WORDS TO DESCRIBE MY DAY

STRUGGLES

HIGHLIGHT OF MY DAY

DAILY ACCOMPLISHMENTS

DAILY *Reflection*

HOW I FEEL TODAY

MY GREATEST CHALLENGE

MOOD TRACKER:

MORNING:

EVENING:

I FELT HAPPY WHEN:

I FELT EXCITED WHEN:

I FELT ENERGIZED WHEN:

Today's Highlights

What I'm Grateful For Today

DAILY *Awareness*

MONTH:

M	T	W	T	F	S	S
☐	☐	☐	☐	☐	☐	☐

HOW I'M FEELING TODAY

3 WORDS TO DESCRIBE MY DAY

STRUGGLES

HIGHLIGHT OF MY DAY

DAILY ACCOMPLISHMENTS

DATE:

DAILY *Reflection*

HOW I FEEL TODAY

MY GREATEST CHALLENGE

MOOD TRACKER:

MORNING:

EVENING:

I FELT HAPPY WHEN:

I FELT EXCITED WHEN:

I FELT ENERGIZED WHEN:

Today's Highlights

What I'm Grateful For Today

DAILY *Awareness*

MONTH:

M	T	W	T	F	S	S
☐	☐	☐	☐	☐	☐	☐

HOW I'M FEELING TODAY

3 WORDS TO DESCRIBE MY DAY

STRUGGLES

HIGHLIGHT OF MY DAY

DAILY ACCOMPLISHMENTS

DAILY *Reflection*

DATE:

HOW I FEEL TODAY

MY GREATEST CHALLENGE

MOOD TRACKER:

MORNING:

EVENING:

I FELT HAPPY WHEN:

I FELT EXCITED WHEN:

I FELT ENERGIZED WHEN:

Today's Highlights

What I'm Grateful For Today

DAILY *Awareness*

MONTH:

M	T	W	T	F	S	S
☐	☐	☐	☐	☐	☐	☐

HOW I'M FEELING TODAY

3 WORDS TO DESCRIBE MY DAY

STRUGGLES

HIGHLIGHT OF MY DAY

DAILY ACCOMPLISHMENTS

DATE:

DAILY *Reflection*

HOW I FEEL TODAY

MY GREATEST CHALLENGE

MOOD TRACKER:

MORNING:

EVENING:

I FELT HAPPY WHEN:

I FELT EXCITED WHEN:

I FELT ENERGIZED WHEN:

Today's Highlights

What I'm Grateful For Today

DAILY *Awareness*

MONTH:

M	T	W	T	F	S	S
☐	☐	☐	☐	☐	☐	☐

HOW I'M FEELING TODAY

3 WORDS TO DESCRIBE MY DAY

STRUGGLES

HIGHLIGHT OF MY DAY

DAILY ACCOMPLISHMENTS

DAILY *Reflection*

HOW I FEEL TODAY

MY GREATEST CHALLENGE

MOOD TRACKER:

MORNING:

EVENING:

I FELT HAPPY WHEN:

I FELT EXCITED WHEN:

I FELT ENERGIZED WHEN:

Today's Highlights

What I'm Grateful For Today

ANXIETY *Tracker*

Document the days when you experienced anxiety. This page includes a 3-week tracker.

ANXIETY LEVELS (1-MILD, 10 SEVERE)

MON	01	02	03	04	05	06	07	08	09	10	11	12
TUE	01	02	03	04	05	06	07	08	09	10	11	12
WED	01	02	03	04	05	06	07	08	09	10	11	12
THU	01	02	03	04	05	06	07	08	09	10	11	12
FRI	01	02	03	04	05	06	07	08	09	10	11	12
SAT	01	02	03	04	05	06	07	08	09	10	11	12
SUN	01	02	03	04	05	06	07	08	09	10	11	12
MON	01	02	03	04	05	06	07	08	09	10	11	12
TUE	01	02	03	04	05	06	07	08	09	10	11	12
WED	01	02	03	04	05	06	07	08	09	10	11	12
THU	01	02	03	04	05	06	07	08	09	10	11	12
FRI	01	02	03	04	05	06	07	08	09	10	11	12
SAT	01	02	03	04	05	06	07	08	09	10	11	12
SUN	01	02	03	04	05	06	07	08	09	10	11	12
MON	01	02	03	04	05	06	07	08	09	10	11	12
TUE	01	02	03	04	05	06	07	08	09	10	11	12
WED	01	02	03	04	05	06	07	08	09	10	11	12
THU	01	02	03	04	05	06	07	08	09	10	11	12
FRI	01	02	03	04	05	06	07	08	09	10	11	12
SAT	01	02	03	04	05	06	07	08	09	10	11	12
SUN	01	02	03	04	05	06	07	08	09	10	11	12

NOTES:

DATE I STARTED TRACKING:

DEPRESSION *Tracker*

Document the days when you experienced depression. This page includes a 3-week tracker.

DEPRESSION LEVELS (1-MILD, 10 SEVERE)

MON	01	02	03	04	05	06	07	08	09	10	11	12
TUE	01	02	03	04	05	06	07	08	09	10	11	12
WED	01	02	03	04	05	06	07	08	09	10	11	12
THU	01	02	03	04	05	06	07	08	09	10	11	12
FRI	01	02	03	04	05	06	07	08	09	10	11	12
SAT	01	02	03	04	05	06	07	08	09	10	11	12
SUN	01	02	03	04	05	06	07	08	09	10	11	12
MON	01	02	03	04	05	06	07	08	09	10	11	12
TUE	01	02	03	04	05	06	07	08	09	10	11	12
WED	01	02	03	04	05	06	07	08	09	10	11	12
THU	01	02	03	04	05	06	07	08	09	10	11	12
FRI	01	02	03	04	05	06	07	08	09	10	11	12
SAT	01	02	03	04	05	06	07	08	09	10	11	12
SUN	01	02	03	04	05	06	07	08	09	10	11	12
MON	01	02	03	04	05	06	07	08	09	10	11	12
TUE	01	02	03	04	05	06	07	08	09	10	11	12
WED	01	02	03	04	05	06	07	08	09	10	11	12
THU	01	02	03	04	05	06	07	08	09	10	11	12
FRI	01	02	03	04	05	06	07	08	09	10	11	12
SAT	01	02	03	04	05	06	07	08	09	10	11	12
SUN	01	02	03	04	05	06	07	08	09	10	11	12

NOTES:

DATE I STARTED TRACKING:

DAILY *Awareness*

MONTH:

M T W T F S S
☐ ☐ ☐ ☐ ☐ ☐ ☐

HOW I'M FEELING TODAY

3 WORDS TO DESCRIBE MY DAY

STRUGGLES

HIGHLIGHT OF MY DAY

DAILY ACCOMPLISHMENTS

POST *Therapy Chart*

DATE:

SUMMARY/OVERVIEW OF THERAPY SESSION

WHAT WE DISCUSSED

HOW IT MADE ME FEEL

WHAT I LEARNED

WHAT I WANT TO DISCUSS NEXT

Rate your session to keep track of progress.

SESSION SCORE

THOUGHTS *Tracker*

MONITORING YOUR THOUGHTS & FEELINGS

MONDAY'S THOUGHTS

TUESDAY'S THOUGHTS

WEDNESDAY'S THOUGHTS

THURSDAY'S THOUGHTS

FRIDAY'S THOUGHTS

SATURDAY'S THOUGHTS

SUNDAY'S THOUGHTS

WEEKLY *Assessment*

	SLEEP	MOOD	POSITIVES	NEGATIVES
MONDAY				
TUESDAY				
WEDNESDAY				
THURSDAY				
FRIDAY				
SATURADY				
SUNDAY				

WEEKLY *Reflections*

Monday

Tuesday

Wednesday

Thursday

Friday

Saturday

Sunday

DATE:

DAILY *Reflection*

HOW I FEEL TODAY

MY GREATEST CHALLENGE

MOOD TRACKER:

MORNING:

EVENING:

I FELT HAPPY WHEN:

I FELT EXCITED WHEN:

I FELT ENERGIZED WHEN:

Today's Highlights

What I'm Grateful For Today

DAILY Awareness

MONTH:

M T W T F S S
☐ ☐ ☐ ☐ ☐ ☐ ☐

HOW I'M FEELING TODAY

3 WORDS TO DESCRIBE MY DAY

STRUGGLES

HIGHLIGHT OF MY DAY

DAILY ACCOMPLISHMENTS

DAILY *Reflection*

HOW I FEEL TODAY

MY GREATEST CHALLENGE

MOOD TRACKER:

MORNING:

EVENING:

I FELT HAPPY WHEN:

I FELT EXCITED WHEN:

I FELT ENERGIZED WHEN:

Today's Highlights

What I'm Grateful For Today

DAILY *Awareness*

MONTH:

M	T	W	T	F	S	S
☐	☐	☐	☐	☐	☐	☐

HOW I'M FEELING TODAY

3 WORDS TO DESCRIBE MY DAY

STRUGGLES

HIGHLIGHT OF MY DAY

DAILY ACCOMPLISHMENTS

DAILY Reflection

DATE:

HOW I FEEL TODAY

MY GREATEST CHALLENGE

MOOD TRACKER:

MORNING:

EVENING:

I FELT HAPPY WHEN:

I FELT EXCITED WHEN:

I FELT ENERGIZED WHEN:

Today's Highlights

What I'm Grateful For Today

DAILY *Awareness*

MONTH:

M	T	W	T	F	S	S
☐	☐	☐	☐	☐	☐	☐

HOW I'M FEELING TODAY

3 WORDS TO DESCRIBE MY DAY

STRUGGLES

HIGHLIGHT OF MY DAY

DAILY ACCOMPLISHMENTS

DATE:

DAILY *Reflection*

HOW I FEEL TODAY

MY GREATEST CHALLENGE

MOOD TRACKER:

MORNING:

EVENING:

I FELT HAPPY WHEN:

I FELT EXCITED WHEN:

I FELT ENERGIZED WHEN:

Today's Highlights

What I'm Grateful For Today

DAILY *Awareness*

MONTH:

M	T	W	T	F	S	S
☐	☐	☐	☐	☐	☐	☐

HOW I'M FEELING TODAY

3 WORDS TO DESCRIBE MY DAY

STRUGGLES

HIGHLIGHT OF MY DAY

DAILY ACCOMPLISHMENTS

DATE:

DAILY Reflection

HOW I FEEL TODAY

MY GREATEST CHALLENGE

MOOD TRACKER:

MORNING:

EVENING:

I FELT HAPPY WHEN:

I FELT EXCITED WHEN:

I FELT ENERGIZED WHEN:

Today's Highlights

What I'm Grateful For Today

DAILY *Awareness*

MONTH:

M	T	W	T	F	S	S
☐	☐	☐	☐	☐	☐	☐

HOW I'M FEELING TODAY

3 WORDS TO DESCRIBE MY DAY

STRUGGLES

HIGHLIGHT OF MY DAY

DAILY ACCOMPLISHMENTS

DAILY Reflection

HOW I FEEL TODAY

MY GREATEST CHALLENGE

MOOD TRACKER:

MORNING:

EVENING:

I FELT HAPPY WHEN:

I FELT EXCITED WHEN:

I FELT ENERGIZED WHEN:

Today's Highlights

What I'm Grateful For Today

DAILY *Awareness*

MONTH:

M	T	W	T	F	S	S
☐	☐	☐	☐	☐	☐	☐

HOW I'M FEELING TODAY

3 WORDS TO DESCRIBE MY DAY

STRUGGLES

HIGHLIGHT OF MY DAY

DAILY ACCOMPLISHMENTS

DATE:

DAILY *Reflection*

HOW I FEEL TODAY

MY GREATEST CHALLENGE

MOOD TRACKER:

MORNING:

EVENING:

I FELT HAPPY WHEN:

I FELT EXCITED WHEN:

I FELT ENERGIZED WHEN:

Today's Highlights

What I'm Grateful For Today

DAILY *Awareness*

MONTH:

M T W T F S S
☐ ☐ ☐ ☐ ☐ ☐ ☐

HOW I'M FEELING TODAY

3 WORDS TO DESCRIBE MY DAY

STRUGGLES

HIGHLIGHT OF MY DAY

DAILY ACCOMPLISHMENTS

POST *Therapy Chart*

DATE:

SUMMARY/OVERVIEW OF THERAPY SESSION

WHAT WE DISCUSSED

HOW IT MADE ME FEEL

WHAT I LEARNED

WHAT I WANT TO DISCUSS NEXT

Rate your session to keep track of progress.

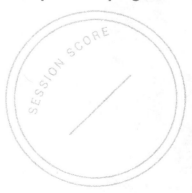

SESSION SCORE

THOUGHTS *Tracker*

MONITORING YOUR THOUGHTS & FEELINGS

MONDAY'S THOUGHTS

TUESDAY'S THOUGHTS

WEDNESDAY'S THOUGHTS

THURSDAY'S THOUGHTS

FRIDAY'S THOUGHTS

SATURDAY'S THOUGHTS

SUNDAY'S THOUGHTS

WEEKLY *Assessment*

	SLEEP	MOOD	POSITIVES	NEGATIVES
MONDAY				
TUESDAY				
WEDNESDAY				
THURSDAY				
FRIDAY				
SATURDAY				
SUNDAY				

WEEKLY *Reflections*

Monday

Tuesday

Wednesday

Thursday

Friday

Saturday

Sunday

DAILY *Reflection*

HOW I FEEL TODAY

MY GREATEST CHALLENGE

MOOD TRACKER:

MORNING:

EVENING:

I FELT HAPPY WHEN:

I FELT EXCITED WHEN:

I FELT ENERGIZED WHEN:

Today's Highlights

What I'm Grateful For Today

DAILY *Awareness*

MONTH:

M	T	W	T	F	S	S
☐	☐	☐	☐	☐	☐	☐

HOW I'M FEELING TODAY

3 WORDS TO DESCRIBE MY DAY

STRUGGLES

HIGHLIGHT OF MY DAY

DAILY ACCOMPLISHMENTS

DATE:

DAILY *Reflection*

HOW I FEEL TODAY

MY GREATEST CHALLENGE

MOOD TRACKER:

MORNING:

EVENING:

I FELT HAPPY WHEN:

I FELT EXCITED WHEN:

I FELT ENERGIZED WHEN:

Today's Highlights

What I'm Grateful For Today

DAILY *Awareness*

MONTH:

M   T   W   T   F   S   S

☐ ☐ ☐ ☐ ☐ ☐ ☐

HOW I'M FEELING TODAY

3 WORDS TO DESCRIBE MY DAY

STRUGGLES

HIGHLIGHT OF MY DAY

DAILY ACCOMPLISHMENTS

DATE:

DAILY *Reflection*

HOW I FEEL TODAY

MY GREATEST CHALLENGE

MOOD TRACKER:

MORNING:

EVENING:

I FELT HAPPY WHEN:

I FELT EXCITED WHEN:

I FELT ENERGIZED WHEN:

Today's Highlights

What I'm Grateful For Today

DAILY Awareness

MONTH:

M   T   W   T   F   S   S
☐   ☐   ☐   ☐   ☐   ☐   ☐

HOW I'M FEELING TODAY

3 WORDS TO DESCRIBE MY DAY

STRUGGLES

HIGHLIGHT OF MY DAY

DAILY ACCOMPLISHMENTS

DATE:

DAILY *Reflection*

HOW I FEEL TODAY

MY GREATEST CHALLENGE

MOOD TRACKER:

MORNING:

EVENING:

I FELT HAPPY WHEN:

I FELT EXCITED WHEN:

I FELT ENERGIZED WHEN:

Today's Highlights

What I'm Grateful For Today

DAILY *Awareness*

MONTH:

M	T	W	T	F	S	S
☐	☐	☐	☐	☐	☐	☐

HOW I'M FEELING TODAY

3 WORDS TO DESCRIBE MY DAY

STRUGGLES

HIGHLIGHT OF MY DAY

DAILY ACCOMPLISHMENTS

DATE:

DAILY *Reflection*

HOW I FEEL TODAY

MY GREATEST CHALLENGE

MOOD TRACKER:

MORNING:

EVENING:

I FELT HAPPY WHEN:

I FELT EXCITED WHEN:

I FELT ENERGIZED WHEN:

Today's Highlights

What I'm Grateful For Today

DAILY *Awareness*

MONTH:

M	T	W	T	F	S	S
☐	☐	☐	☐	☐	☐	☐

HOW I'M FEELING TODAY

3 WORDS TO DESCRIBE MY DAY

STRUGGLES

HIGHLIGHT OF MY DAY

DAILY ACCOMPLISHMENTS

DATE:

DAILY *Reflection*

HOW I FEEL TODAY

MY GREATEST CHALLENGE

MOOD TRACKER:

MORNING:

EVENING:

I FELT HAPPY WHEN:

I FELT EXCITED WHEN:

I FELT ENERGIZED WHEN:

Today's Highlights

What I'm Grateful For Today

DAILY *Awareness*

MONTH:

M	T	W	T	F	S	S
☐	☐	☐	☐	☐	☐	☐

HOW I'M FEELING TODAY

3 WORDS TO DESCRIBE MY DAY

STRUGGLES

HIGHLIGHT OF MY DAY

DAILY ACCOMPLISHMENTS

DAILY *Reflection*

HOW I FEEL TODAY

MY GREATEST CHALLENGE

MOOD TRACKER:

MORNING:

EVENING:

I FELT HAPPY WHEN:

I FELT EXCITED WHEN:

I FELT ENERGIZED WHEN:

Today's Highlights

What I'm Grateful For Today

DAILY *Awareness*

MONTH:

M	T	W	T	F	S	S
☐	☐	☐	☐	☐	☐	☐

HOW I'M FEELING TODAY

3 WORDS TO DESCRIBE MY DAY

STRUGGLES

HIGHLIGHT OF MY DAY

DAILY ACCOMPLISHMENTS

POST *Therapy Chart*

DATE:

SUMMARY/OVERVIEW OF THERAPY SESSION

WHAT WE DISCUSSED

HOW IT MADE ME FEEL

WHAT I LEARNED

WHAT I WANT TO DISCUSS NEXT

Rate your session to keep track of progress.

SESSION SCORE

THOUGHTS *Tracker*

MONDAY'S THOUGHTS

TUESDAY'S THOUGHTS

WEDNESDAY'S THOUGHTS

THURSDAY'S THOUGHTS

FRIDAY'S THOUGHTS

SATURDAY'S THOUGHTS

SUNDAY'S THOUGHTS

WEEKLY *Assessment*

	SLEEP	MOOD	POSITIVES	NEGATIVES
MONDAY				
TUESDAY				
WEDNESDAY				
THURSDAY				
FRIDAY				
SATURADY				
SUNDAY				

WEEKLY *Reflections*

Monday

Tuesday

Wednesday

Thursday

Friday

Saturday

Sunday

DAILY *Reflection*

HOW I FEEL TODAY

MY GREATEST CHALLENGE

MOOD TRACKER:

MORNING:

EVENING:

I FELT HAPPY WHEN:

I FELT EXCITED WHEN:

I FELT ENERGIZED WHEN:

Today's Highlights

What I'm Grateful For Today

DAILY *Awareness*

MONTH:

M T W T F S S
☐ ☐ ☐ ☐ ☐ ☐ ☐

HOW I'M FEELING TODAY

3 WORDS TO DESCRIBE MY DAY

STRUGGLES

HIGHLIGHT OF MY DAY

DAILY ACCOMPLISHMENTS

DAILY *Reflection*

HOW I FEEL TODAY

MY GREATEST CHALLENGE

MOOD TRACKER:

MORNING:

EVENING:

I FELT HAPPY WHEN:

I FELT EXCITED WHEN:

I FELT ENERGIZED WHEN:

Today's Highlights

What I'm Grateful For Today

DAILY *Awareness*

MONTH:

M T W T F S S
☐ ☐ ☐ ☐ ☐ ☐ ☐

HOW I'M FEELING TODAY

3 WORDS TO DESCRIBE MY DAY

STRUGGLES

HIGHLIGHT OF MY DAY

DAILY ACCOMPLISHMENTS

DATE:

DAILY *Reflection*

HOW I FEEL TODAY

MY GREATEST CHALLENGE

MOOD TRACKER:

MORNING:

EVENING:

I FELT HAPPY WHEN:

I FELT EXCITED WHEN:

I FELT ENERGIZED WHEN:

Today's Highlights

What I'm Grateful For Today

DAILY *Awareness*

MONTH:

M	T	W	T	F	S	S
☐	☐	☐	☐	☐	☐	☐

HOW I'M FEELING TODAY

3 WORDS TO DESCRIBE MY DAY

STRUGGLES

HIGHLIGHT OF MY DAY

DAILY ACCOMPLISHMENTS

DATE:

DAILY *Reflection*

HOW I FEEL TODAY

MY GREATEST CHALLENGE

MOOD TRACKER:

MORNING:

EVENING:

I FELT HAPPY WHEN:

I FELT EXCITED WHEN:

I FELT ENERGIZED WHEN:

Today's Highlights

What I'm Grateful For Today

DAILY *Awareness*

MONTH:

M	T	W	T	F	S	S
☐	☐	☐	☐	☐	☐	☐

HOW I'M FEELING TODAY

3 WORDS TO DESCRIBE MY DAY

STRUGGLES

HIGHLIGHT OF MY DAY

DAILY ACCOMPLISHMENTS

DATE:

DAILY *Reflection*

HOW I FEEL TODAY

MY GREATEST CHALLENGE

MOOD TRACKER:

MORNING:

EVENING:

I FELT HAPPY WHEN:

I FELT EXCITED WHEN:

I FELT ENERGIZED WHEN:

Today's Highlights

What I'm Grateful For Today

DAILY *Awareness*

MONTH:

M T W T F S S
☐ ☐ ☐ ☐ ☐ ☐ ☐

HOW I'M FEELING TODAY

3 WORDS TO DESCRIBE MY DAY

STRUGGLES

HIGHLIGHT OF MY DAY

DAILY ACCOMPLISHMENTS

DATE:

DAILY *Reflection*

HOW I FEEL TODAY

MY GREATEST CHALLENGE

MOOD TRACKER:

MORNING:

EVENING:

I FELT HAPPY WHEN:

I FELT EXCITED WHEN:

I FELT ENERGIZED WHEN:

Today's Highlights

What I'm Grateful For Today

DAILY *Awareness*

MONTH:

M T W T F S S

☐ ☐ ☐ ☐ ☐ ☐ ☐

HOW I'M FEELING TODAY

3 WORDS TO DESCRIBE MY DAY

STRUGGLES

HIGHLIGHT OF MY DAY

DAILY ACCOMPLISHMENTS

DATE:

DAILY *Reflection*

HOW I FEEL TODAY

MY GREATEST CHALLENGE

MOOD TRACKER:

MORNING:

EVENING:

I FELT HAPPY WHEN:

I FELT EXCITED WHEN:

I FELT ENERGIZED WHEN:

Today's Highlights

What I'm Grateful For Today

DAILY *Awareness*

MONTH:

M	T	W	T	F	S	S
☐	☐	☐	☐	☐	☐	☐

HOW I'M FEELING TODAY

3 WORDS TO DESCRIBE MY DAY

STRUGGLES

HIGHLIGHT OF MY DAY

DAILY ACCOMPLISHMENTS

POST *Therapy Chart*

DATE:

SUMMARY/OVERVIEW OF THERAPY SESSION

WHAT WE DISCUSSED

HOW IT MADE ME FEEL

WHAT I LEARNED

WHAT I WANT TO DISCUSS NEXT

Rate your session to keep track of progress.

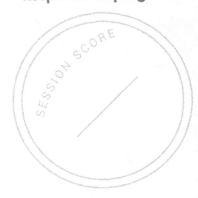

SESSION SCORE

THOUGHTS *Tracker*

MONITORING YOUR THOUGHTS & FEELINGS

MONDAY'S THOUGHTS

TUESDAY'S THOUGHTS

WEDNESDAY'S THOUGHTS

THURSDAY'S THOUGHTS

FRIDAY'S THOUGHTS

SATURDAY'S THOUGHTS

SUNDAY'S THOUGHTS

WEEKLY *Reflections*

Monday

Tuesday

Wednesday

Thursday

Friday

Saturday

Sunday

DAILY Reflection

DATE:

HOW I FEEL TODAY

MY GREATEST CHALLENGE

MOOD TRACKER:

MORNING:

EVENING:

I FELT HAPPY WHEN:

I FELT EXCITED WHEN:

I FELT ENERGIZED WHEN:

Today's Highlights

What I'm Grateful For Today

DAILY *Awareness*

MONTH:

M	T	W	T	F	S	S
☐	☐	☐	☐	☐	☐	☐

HOW I'M FEELING TODAY

3 WORDS TO DESCRIBE MY DAY

STRUGGLES

HIGHLIGHT OF MY DAY

DAILY ACCOMPLISHMENTS

DATE:

DAILY *Reflection*

HOW I FEEL TODAY

MY GREATEST CHALLENGE

MOOD TRACKER:

MORNING:

EVENING:

I FELT HAPPY WHEN:

I FELT EXCITED WHEN:

I FELT ENERGIZED WHEN:

Today's Highlights

What I'm Grateful For Today

DAILY *Awareness*

MONTH:

M	T	W	T	F	S	S
☐	☐	☐	☐	☐	☐	☐

HOW I'M FEELING TODAY

3 WORDS TO DESCRIBE MY DAY

STRUGGLES

HIGHLIGHT OF MY DAY

DAILY ACCOMPLISHMENTS

DAILY *Reflection*

HOW I FEEL TODAY

MY GREATEST CHALLENGE

MOOD TRACKER:

MORNING:

EVENING:

I FELT HAPPY WHEN:

I FELT EXCITED WHEN:

I FELT ENERGIZED WHEN:

Today's Highlights

What I'm Grateful For Today

DAILY *Awareness*

MONTH:

M	T	W	T	F	S	S
☐	☐	☐	☐	☐	☐	☐

HOW I'M FEELING TODAY

3 WORDS TO DESCRIBE MY DAY

STRUGGLES

HIGHLIGHT OF MY DAY

DAILY ACCOMPLISHMENTS

DATE:

DAILY *Reflection*

HOW I FEEL TODAY

MY GREATEST CHALLENGE

MOOD TRACKER:

MORNING:

EVENING:

I FELT HAPPY WHEN:

I FELT EXCITED WHEN:

I FELT ENERGIZED WHEN:

Today's Highlights

What I'm Grateful For Today

DAILY *Awareness*

MONTH:

M T W T F S S
☐ ☐ ☐ ☐ ☐ ☐ ☐

HOW I'M FEELING TODAY

3 WORDS TO DESCRIBE MY DAY

STRUGGLES

HIGHLIGHT OF MY DAY

DAILY ACCOMPLISHMENTS

DAILY *Reflection*

HOW I FEEL TODAY

MY GREATEST CHALLENGE

MOOD TRACKER:

MORNING:

EVENING:

I FELT HAPPY WHEN:

I FELT EXCITED WHEN:

I FELT ENERGIZED WHEN:

Today's Highlights

What I'm Grateful For Today

DAILY *Awareness*

MONTH: _____

M   T   W   T   F   S   S

☐   ☐   ☐   ☐   ☐   ☐   ☐

HOW I'M FEELING TODAY

3 WORDS TO DESCRIBE MY DAY

STRUGGLES

HIGHLIGHT OF MY DAY

DAILY ACCOMPLISHMENTS

DAILY *Reflection*

HOW I FEEL TODAY

MY GREATEST CHALLENGE

MOOD TRACKER:

MORNING:

EVENING:

I FELT HAPPY WHEN:

I FELT EXCITED WHEN:

I FELT ENERGIZED WHEN:

Today's Highlights

What I'm Grateful For Today

DAILY *Awareness*

MONTH:

M	T	W	T	F	S	S
☐	☐	☐	☐	☐	☐	☐

HOW I'M FEELING TODAY

3 WORDS TO DESCRIBE MY DAY

STRUGGLES

HIGHLIGHT OF MY DAY

DAILY ACCOMPLISHMENTS

DAILY *Reflection*

DATE:

HOW I FEEL TODAY

MY GREATEST CHALLENGE

MOOD TRACKER:

MORNING:

EVENING:

I FELT HAPPY WHEN:

I FELT EXCITED WHEN:

I FELT ENERGIZED WHEN:

Today's Highlights

What I'm Grateful For Today

DAILY *Awareness*

MONTH:

M T W T F S S
☐ ☐ ☐ ☐ ☐ ☐ ☐

HOW I'M FEELING TODAY

3 WORDS TO DESCRIBE MY DAY

STRUGGLES

HIGHLIGHT OF MY DAY

DAILY ACCOMPLISHMENTS

POST *Therapy Chart*

DATE:

SUMMARY/OVERVIEW OF THERAPY SESSION

WHAT WE DISCUSSED

HOW IT MADE ME FEEL

WHAT I LEARNED

WHAT I WANT TO DISCUSS NEXT

Rate your session to keep track of progress.

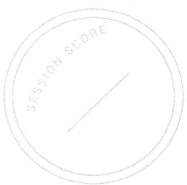

SESSION SCORE

THOUGHTS *Tracker*

MONITORING YOUR THOUGHTS & FEELINGS

MONDAY'S THOUGHTS

TUESDAY'S THOUGHTS

WEDNESDAY'S THOUGHTS

THURSDAY'S THOUGHTS

FRIDAY'S THOUGHTS

SATURDAY'S THOUGHTS

SUNDAY'S THOUGHTS

WEEKLY *Reflections*

Monday

Tuesday

Wednesday

Thursday

Friday

Saturday

Sunday

DATE:

DAILY *Reflection*

HOW I FEEL TODAY

MY GREATEST CHALLENGE

MOOD TRACKER:

MORNING:

EVENING:

I FELT HAPPY WHEN:

I FELT EXCITED WHEN:

I FELT ENERGIZED WHEN:

Today's Highlights

What I'm Grateful For Today

DAILY *Awareness*

MONTH:

M	T	W	T	F	S	S
☐	☐	☐	☐	☐	☐	☐

HOW I'M FEELING TODAY

3 WORDS TO DESCRIBE MY DAY

STRUGGLES

HIGHLIGHT OF MY DAY

DAILY ACCOMPLISHMENTS

DATE:

DAILY *Reflection*

HOW I FEEL TODAY

MY GREATEST CHALLENGE

MOOD TRACKER:

MORNING:

EVENING:

I FELT HAPPY WHEN:

I FELT EXCITED WHEN:

I FELT ENERGIZED WHEN:

Today's Highlights

What I'm Grateful For Today

DAILY *Awareness*

MONTH:

M T W T F S S

□ □ □ □ □ □ □

HOW I'M FEELING TODAY

3 WORDS TO DESCRIBE MY DAY

STRUGGLES

HIGHLIGHT OF MY DAY

DAILY ACCOMPLISHMENTS

DATE:

DAILY *Reflection*

HOW I FEEL TODAY

MY GREATEST CHALLENGE

MOOD TRACKER:

MORNING:

EVENING:

I FELT HAPPY WHEN:

I FELT EXCITED WHEN:

I FELT ENERGIZED WHEN:

Today's Highlights

What I'm Grateful For Today

DAILY *Awareness*

MONTH:

M T W T F S S
☐ ☐ ☐ ☐ ☐ ☐ ☐

HOW I'M FEELING TODAY

3 WORDS TO DESCRIBE MY DAY

STRUGGLES

HIGHLIGHT OF MY DAY

DAILY ACCOMPLISHMENTS

DATE:

DAILY *Reflection*

HOW I FEEL TODAY

MY GREATEST CHALLENGE

MOOD TRACKER:

MORNING:

EVENING:

I FELT HAPPY WHEN:

I FELT EXCITED WHEN:

I FELT ENERGIZED WHEN:

Today's Highlights

What I'm Grateful For Today

DAILY *Awareness*

MONTH:

M   T   W   T   F   S   S
☐   ☐   ☐   ☐   ☐   ☐   ☐

HOW I'M FEELING TODAY

3 WORDS TO DESCRIBE MY DAY

STRUGGLES

HIGHLIGHT OF MY DAY

DAILY ACCOMPLISHMENTS

DATE:

DAILY *Reflection*

HOW I FEEL TODAY

MY GREATEST CHALLENGE

MOOD TRACKER:

MORNING:

EVENING:

I FELT HAPPY WHEN:

I FELT EXCITED WHEN:

I FELT ENERGIZED WHEN:

Today's Highlights

What I'm Grateful For Today

DAILY *Awareness*

MONTH:

M	T	W	T	F	S	S
☐	☐	☐	☐	☐	☐	☐

HOW I'M FEELING TODAY

3 WORDS TO DESCRIBE MY DAY

STRUGGLES

HIGHLIGHT OF MY DAY

DAILY ACCOMPLISHMENTS

DATE:

DAILY *Reflection*

HOW I FEEL TODAY

MY GREATEST CHALLENGE

MOOD TRACKER:

MORNING:

EVENING:

I FELT HAPPY WHEN:

I FELT EXCITED WHEN:

I FELT ENERGIZED WHEN:

Today's Highlights

What I'm Grateful For Today

DAILY *Awareness*

MONTH:

M T W T F S S
☐ ☐ ☐ ☐ ☐ ☐ ☐

HOW I'M FEELING TODAY

3 WORDS TO DESCRIBE MY DAY

STRUGGLES

HIGHLIGHT OF MY DAY

DAILY ACCOMPLISHMENTS

DATE:

DAILY *Reflection*

HOW I FEEL TODAY

MY GREATEST CHALLENGE

MOOD TRACKER:

MORNING:

EVENING:

I FELT HAPPY WHEN:

I FELT EXCITED WHEN:

I FELT ENERGIZED WHEN:

Today's Highlights

What I'm Grateful For Today

DAILY *Awareness*

MONTH:

M T W T F S S

HOW I'M FEELING TODAY

3 WORDS TO DESCRIBE MY DAY

STRUGGLES

HIGHLIGHT OF MY DAY

DAILY ACCOMPLISHMENTS

POST *Therapy Chart*

DATE:

SUMMARY/OVERVIEW OF THERAPY SESSION

WHAT WE DISCUSSED

HOW IT MADE ME FEEL

WHAT I LEARNED

WHAT I WANT TO DISCUSS NEXT

Rate your session to keep track of progress.

SESSION SCORE

THOUGHTS Tracker

MONDAY'S THOUGHTS

TUESDAY'S THOUGHTS

WEDNESDAY'S THOUGHTS

THURSDAY'S THOUGHTS

FRIDAY'S THOUGHTS

SATURDAY'S THOUGHTS

SUNDAY'S THOUGHTS

WEEKLY *Reflections*

Monday

Tuesday

Wednesday

Thursday

Friday

Saturday

Sunday